Discovering the Full Spectrum

of Holistic Health: Your

Pathway to Peak Well-Being

By

Dr. Tamiko Coleman

Introduction

This book transcends conventional health wisdom, guiding you towards a realm of holistic well-being that promises not just physical health but a profound transformation of your mind, body, and spirit. Prepare to be enraptured by a holistic experience like no other as you uncover the secrets to unlocking your peak well-being.In a world inundated with health and wellness advice, where myriad paths to well-being beckon, 'Discovering the Full Spectrum of Holistic Health: Your Pathway to Peak Well-Being' emerges as a luminous beacon amidst the vast sea of information. This book is a meticulously crafted, unique, and distinct guide that invites you to embark on a transformative journey like no other.

Imagine a journey that transcends the ordinary, one that ventures far beyond the conventional definitions of health and wellness. As you turn the pages of this book, you'll find yourself on the cusp of a profound exploration, where the very essence of well-being unfurls before your eyes. Holistic health, often misunderstood or misrepresented, takes center stage within these pages. It isn't just about treating symptoms; it's about embracing the full spectrum of your well-being. It delves deep into the interconnectedness of your mind, body, and spirit, offering a comprehensive approach that promises not just physical health but a life brimming with vitality, purpose, and balance.

This book is your trusted guide, your companion on a remarkable journey. It reveals the secrets to unlocking your peak well-being, a state where every facet of your existence aligns harmoniously.

Through an array of insights, practices, and wisdom from experts in the field, you'll discover the intricate web of factors that contribute to your overall health.

Prepare to be captivated as you explore the vibrant tapestry of wellness within these pages. Each chapter is a brushstroke on the canvas of your well-being, painting a vivid picture of possibilities. It beckons you to cultivate mindfulness, nurture your body, and embrace the transformative power of holistic living. In a world often characterized by quick fixes and superficial solutions, this book offers a refreshing departure. It invites you to delve deeper, to consider the full spectrum of your health, and to embark on a journey that promises lasting, profound change. It's not just a book; it's a pathway to becoming the best version of yourself. So, open these pages with anticipation, for within them lies the promise of a life illuminated by the radiant light of holistic health, where well-being is not just a destination but a lifelong journey. Welcome to the beginning of your transformation.

Book Of Contents

Chapter 1
The Mind Body of Connection

The mind-body connection is a profound and intricate phenomenon that has captivated the minds of scholars, scientists, and health practitioners throughout history. It is the intricate interplay between our mental and emotional states and our physical well-being. This connection, often described as the bridge between the conscious and the corporeal, transcends mere philosophical contemplation; it wields profound implications for our health, healing, and overall quality of life.

Historical Perspectives

The recognition of the mind-body connection is not a recent revelation. Ancient civilizations such as China and India were among the first to acknowledge the importance of this connection in maintaining holistic health. In ancient Chinese medicine, the concept of Qi, the vital energy flowing through the body, emphasizes the balance between mental and physical health. Ayurveda, the traditional Indian system of medicine, echoes this sentiment, emphasizing the role of mental and emotional factors in physical well-being. Even the ancient Greek philosophers pondered the duality of the mind and body, setting the stage for centuries of exploration. The concept of the mind-body connection has fascinated philosophers, scholars, and medical practitioners for centuries, shaping our understanding of human health and well-being. Throughout history, various perspectives have emerged, contributing to our evolving comprehension of this intricate relationship.

In ancient Greece, the philosopher Plato proposed the idea of a tripartite soul, consisting of reason, spirit, and appetite. This notion laid the groundwork for later theories on the mind's influence on bodily functions. Aristotle, Plato's student, further explored the connection, emphasizing the importance of balance between mental and physical aspects for overall health. During the Middle Ages, the mind-body connection took on a more mystical dimension. The works of figures like Avicenna and Paracelsus blended philosophy with early medical practices, asserting that emotions and mental states could directly affect one's physical health. The Renaissance era saw a resurgence of interest in human anatomy and the mind-body link. Renowned anatomist Andreas Vesalius challenged prevailing beliefs, paving the way for a more empirical approach to understanding the body's functions. In the 17th century, René Descartes famously proposed a dualistic view, separating the mind and body into distinct entities. While this Cartesian dualism has been influential, it has also sparked debates about the true nature of the mind-body connection. In the 19th century, the emergence of psychology as a distinct field led to a deeper exploration of mental processes and their impact on physical health. Psychosomatic medicine gained prominence, highlighting the role of psychological factors in illness.

Today, modern science continues to unravel the intricacies of the mind-body connection through fields like psychoneuroimmunology and cognitive neuroscience. These perspectives build upon the historical foundations, emphasizing the integral relationship between mental and physical health. Historical perspectives on the mind-body connection have evolved over centuries, from ancient Greece to the modern era. These perspectives have shaped our understanding of the intricate interplay between the mind and body, with ongoing research continually enriching our comprehension of this complex relationship.

Modern Scientific Understanding

In the modern era, scientific research has unraveled some of the intricate mechanisms governing the mind-body connection. The field of psychoneuroimmunology delves deep into the interplay between our thoughts, emotions, and our immune system. It has provided empirical evidence demonstrating how chronic stress can weaken the immune response, making individuals more susceptible to illness. We've come a long way from Descartes' notion of a separate mind and body; we now understand that they are intimately linked.

The placebo effect

The placebo effect is a fascinating phenomenon that underscores the intricate relationship between the mind and the body. It refers to the observable improvement in a patient's condition when they receive a treatment with no active therapeutic ingredients simply because they believe it will work. This phenomenon has profound implications for our understanding of the mind-body connection. At its core, the placebo effect showcases the power of belief and expectation. When a person genuinely believes that a treatment will alleviate their symptoms, their brain can trigger a cascade of physiological responses that mimic the effects of real medication. This includes the release of endorphins, neurotransmitters, and even changes in heart rate and blood pressure. These responses demonstrate that our thoughts and perceptions can have tangible effects on our physical well-being.

The mind-body connection becomes even more evident when we consider the mechanisms behind the placebo effect. Research has shown that various brain regions, such as the prefrontal cortex and the anterior cingulate cortex, play crucial roles in modulating pain perception and other bodily sensations. When a person anticipates relief from their symptoms due to a placebo, these brain regions can be activated, influencing the body's response to pain or illness. Moreover, the placebo effect isn't limited to pain management. It has been observed in various medical conditions, ranging from depression and anxiety to autoimmune disorders and gastrointestinal problems. In some cases, placebos have even elicited objective improvements in physiological markers, such as reduced inflammation or enhanced immune responses. These findings challenge our traditional understanding of how the mind and body interact, emphasizing the importance of psychological factors in physical healing. The placebo effect also raises ethical questions in healthcare. While it can be a valuable tool for symptom relief, it's essential for healthcare professionals to be transparent with their patients about the nature of the treatment they are receiving. Honesty and informed consent are paramount, as harnessing the placebo effect ethically requires a delicate balance between psychological support and genuine medical intervention.The placebo effect highlights the intricate and powerful connection between the mind and body. It demonstrates that our beliefs and expectations can influence our physical health and well-being. As our understanding of the mind-body connection continues to evolve, it opens up new avenues for exploring holistic approaches to healthcare that consider both the psychological and physiological aspects of healing. This is also one of the most remarkable phenomena that illustrate the power of the mind-body connection is the placebo effect. It showcases how the mere belief in receiving treatment, even if it's a sugar pill or a sham procedure, can lead to real physiological changes in the body. This raises profound questions about the role of belief, expectation, and the mind's influence over physical health. The placebo effect not only perplexes researchers but also underscores the importance of the mind in influencing physical outcomes.

Stress and its Impact on Health

The influence of chronic stress on health is a prime example of the mind-body connection in action. Prolonged stress, often fueled by negative thoughts and emotions, has been linked to a host of health issues, ranging from cardiovascular diseases to diabetes and autoimmune disorders. Learning to manage stress through various techniques, including meditation, yoga, and cognitive-behavioral therapy, can have a profound impact on physical health. Understanding the psychological stressors that contribute to chronic diseases is an essential step towards holistic well-being.Stress is a natural response to the demands and challenges of life, but when it becomes chronic or overwhelming, it can have a significant impact on physical and mental health. This write-up explores the various ways in which stress affects our well-being.

Mindfulness and Healing

Mindfulness is a practice that has gained widespread recognition for its profound impact on healing and overall well-being. Rooted in ancient Buddhist traditions, mindfulness has found its place in modern medicine and psychology as a powerful tool for promoting physical, emotional, and mental healing. This chapter explores the concept of mindfulness and its transformative effects on the journey of healing them. This practice encourages individuals to observe their experiences with curiosity and acceptance.

Mindfulness Techniques:

•**Meditation:** Meditation is a cornerstone of mindfulness. It involves sitting in a quiet space, focusing on the breath, bodily sensations, or a specific object of attention. Through regular meditation practice, individuals can enhance their ability to stay present and reduce the impact of stress.

•**Breath Awareness:** Breath awareness isn't just a meditation technique; it's a profound journey into the essence of existence.

Picture this, your breath is the artist's brush, and your consciousness is the canvas. With every mindful inhalation, you paint vibrant colors of vitality, filling your inner world with energy and possibility. Exhalation becomes the space where you release the hues of stress and negativity, leaving behind a canvas of serenity. In this exploration of breath awareness, think of your lungs as the bellows of a mystical forge, fanning the flames of your inner strength. With each breath, you're forging resilience, determination, and clarity, shaping yourself into a resilient warrior of life's challenges. Now, consider your breath as the navigator through the labyrinth of your thoughts. When you sail through the seas of your mind, breath is the gentle breeze that guides your ship safely, steering you away from turbulent waters and toward the tranquil shores of mindfulness. Breath awareness isn't just about inhaling and exhaling; it's about recognizing the symphony of sensations that accompany each breath—the rise and fall of your chest, the subtle rush of air through your nostrils, and the soothing rhythm that dances to your unique tune. As you delve deeper into breath awareness, you may discover that each breath carries a message from your body and soul. It whispers tales of your physical health, emotional well-being, and the secrets of your inner world. Listen closely, for within the whispers of your breath, you may find the wisdom to heal and thrive.

In this unique perspective on breath awareness, you're not merely observing your breath; you're forging a profound connection with the very essence of your existence. You're sculpting the masterpiece of your life, stroke by conscious stroke, with the breath as your guiding brush. So, the next time you embark on the journey of breath awareness, remember that you're not just breathing; you're painting the canvas of your life, forging the sword of your resilience, and sailing the seas of self-discovery. Embrace this practice with reverence, for it holds the key to unlocking the vast treasures hidden within you. A body scan involves mentally moving attention through different parts of the body, noticing any tension or discomfort. This technique helps individuals connect with their physical sensations and release pent-up stress.

- **Stress Reduction:** Mindfulness has been extensively studied for its stress-reducing benefits. By fostering a state of calm and awareness, it can lower cortisol levels, boost the immune system, and reduce the harmful effects of chronic stress on the body.

Pain Management: Mindfulness-based techniques, such as Mindfulness-Based Stress Reduction (MBSR), have been effective in helping individuals manage chronic pain conditions. By changing the perception of pain, it can lead to decreased reliance on pain medications.

Emotional Regulation: Mindfulness empowers individuals to observe their emotions without judgment. This heightened emotional intelligence can lead to improved mood, reduced symptoms of anxiety and depression, and healthier relationships.

- **Enhanced Well-Being:** Beyond healing specific ailments, mindfulness cultivates a sense of overall well-being. It encourages a positive outlook on life, increased resilience, and a greater sense of purpose. In the fast-paced world we live in today, where the demands of life often seem to outweigh the time we have to care for ourselves, the pursuit of enhanced well-being has never been more crucial. This chapter is your passport to a journey of self-discovery, personal growth, and lasting happiness.

Picture a life where you wake up each day feeling invigorated, brimming with positivity, and ready to tackle whatever challenges come your way. Imagine a state of well-being that not only encompasses physical health but also mental clarity, emotional resilience, and a deep sense of purpose. This is the life that awaits you as we delve into the profound dimensions of enhanced well-being. But what exactly is enhanced well-being, and why is it so essential in today's world? Throughout this chapter, we will explore the multifaceted nature of well-being and its profound impact on every aspect of our lives. We will uncover the science behind happiness, the power of mindfulness, and the secrets to maintaining a healthy body and mind. Enhanced well-being isn't a destination; it's a lifelong journey. It's about making conscious choices that lead to a life filled with joy, contentment, and a sense of fulfillment. Whether you're seeking to improve your physical fitness, manage stress, build stronger relationships, or simply find more happiness in your everyday existence, this chapter will be your guide. So, are you ready to embark on this transformative journey towards enhanced well-being? Buckle up, because as we dive into the chapters that follow, you'll discover practical strategies, inspiring stories, and actionable insights that will empower you to take charge of your own well-being and lead a life that truly shines.

Let's begin this extraordinary adventure together!

Once upon a time in a remote mountain village, there lived a young woman named Maya. She was known for her boundless energy, radiant health, and unwavering commitment to well-being. Maya believed in the power of nature to heal and revitalize the human spirit. One day, Maya learned about a legendary hidden waterfall deep within the densest part of the nearby forest. It was said that the water from this waterfall possessed magical properties that could rejuvenate the mind, body, and soul. Determined to experience this extraordinary well-being adventure, Maya set out on a journey.

Armed with her backpack filled with nutritious food, meditation tools, and a journal, Maya embarked on her expedition into the heart of the forest. The journey was treacherous, with dense vegetation, slippery slopes, and unpredictable weather. Along the way, she encountered various challenges that tested her physical and mental strength.

However, Maya's unwavering belief in the power of well-being kept her going. She meditated amidst ancient trees, finding serenity even in the face of adversity. She used her knowledge of healing herbs to treat minor injuries, staying true to her commitment to natural remedies. As Maya ventured deeper into the forest, she faced her greatest challenge yet – a roaring river blocking her path to the hidden waterfall. Undeterred, she used her meditation techniques to connect with the elements. In a moment of transcendence, she summoned the strength to navigate the river safely.

Finally, after days of tireless trekking, Maya reached the hidden waterfall. The sight was awe-inspiring – crystal-clear water cascading down moss-covered rocks, surrounded by vibrant flora. Maya immersed herself in the rejuvenating waters, feeling a surge of vitality and well-being like never before. She meditated by the waterfall, documenting her experience in her journal. Maya's extraordinary adventure not only transformed her own well-being but also inspired the people of her village. She shared her journey and the importance of connecting with nature and inner peace. Her village began to prioritize well-being, embracing the healing power of their natural surroundings. Maya's adventure became a legend, passed down through generations, a reminder of the extraordinary well-being that can be found in the heart of nature and within ourselves.

- **Healing Trauma:** Mindfulness can be a valuable tool in the healing process for those who have experienced trauma. It helps individuals safely revisit their experiences and develop coping strategies.

Mindfulness is a profound practice that fosters healing on multiple levels—physical, emotional, and mental. Its non-invasive nature and accessibility make it a valuable addition to conventional healthcare and therapy. Whether you are seeking relief from stress, pain, or emotional turmoil, incorporating mindfulness into your life can be a transformative journey towards healing and improved well-being. It's a practice that invites you to embrace the present moment and, in doing so, find the path to healing and inner peace.

Chapter 2

Nourishing Your Body: Nutrition and Diet

In today's fast-paced world, the importance of nourishing our bodies through proper nutrition and diet cannot be overstated. Our bodies are intricate machines, and the fuel we provide them plays a critical role in our overall health, well-being, and longevity. This chapter is your guide to understanding the fundamental principles of nutrition and diet, empowering you to make informed choices that will have a profound impact on your life.

Section 1: The Basics of Nutrition

The Building Blocks of Nutrition: Let start by explaining macronutrients (carbohydrates, proteins, and fats) and micronutrients (vitamins and minerals) and their importance in maintaining health. In a world where health is the most precious asset, understanding the very foundation of well-being is paramount. Welcome to "The Building Blocks of Nutrition," a chapter that unveils the secrets to a vibrant and wholesome life through the power of food. In this enlightening journey, we delve deep into the very essence of nutrition, exploring the fundamental elements that fuel our bodies and minds. Just as a sturdy house requires a strong foundation, our bodies too demand the right building blocks for optimal functioning. In the opening pages, we'll discover the magic of macronutrients – the proteins, carbohydrates, and fats that serve as the cornerstone of our diets. Explore how each of these macronutrients plays a vital role in shaping our health and well-being, and learn how to strike the perfect balance to unlock your body's full potential.

But our exploration doesn't end there. We'll venture into the fascinating world of micronutrients, where vitamins and minerals are the unsung heroes, tirelessly supporting our body's intricate systems. Uncover the unique role that each of these micronutrients plays and how they contribute to your vitality.

As we journey through "The Building Blocks of Nutrition," you'll also gain insights into the importance of hydration, fiber, and antioxidants. These lesser-known elements are like the hidden treasures in your nutritional arsenal, waiting to be unlocked for a healthier you.

Prepare to be captivated by the stories of real-life individuals who have transformed their lives through the wisdom of nutrition. Their inspiring journeys will serve as beacons of hope and motivation, guiding you towards making informed choices for a healthier, more fulfilling life. This chapter isn't just a collection of facts; it's a practical guide to embracing a balanced and nourishing diet. We'll provide you with tips, recipes, and expert advice to help you implement these nutrition building blocks into your daily routine.

"The Building Blocks of Nutrition" is more than just a chapter; it's your roadmap to a healthier, happier life So, let's embark on this transformative journey together and discover the profound impact that nutrition can have on your life.

Macronutrients:

Macronutrients, the vital nutrients our bodies demand in substantial amounts for optimal operation, furnish the energy necessary for daily tasks and compose the cornerstone of our nutritional intake. These fundamental macronutrients encompass carbohydrates, proteins, and fats.

Carbohydrates: Carbohydrates stand as the body's principal energy supplier, existing in two distinct types: simple carbohydrates (sugars) and complex carbohydrates (starches and fibers). Simple sugars deliver rapid energy bursts, whereas complex carbs release energy in a gradual, sustained manner, serving as a fundamental element for both cognitive functioning and overall physiological activities.

Proteins: Proteins are the body's building blocks, crucial for the growth, repair, and maintenance of tissues. They play a pivotal role in forming enzymes, hormones, and antibodies. Protein-rich foods help build muscle, maintain healthy skin, and support the immune system.

Fats: Dietary fats are often misunderstood. They are essential for various bodily functions, including cell structure, hormone production, and the absorption of fat-soluble vitamins (like A, D, E, and K). Nutrient-rich fats, like the ones present in avocados, nuts, and olive oil, play a pivotal role in maintaining our well-being.

Micronutrients:

Micronutrients are nutrients required in smaller quantities but are no less critical for our well-being. They include vitamins and minerals, and they are involved in numerous biochemical processes that keep our bodies functioning optimally.

Vitamins: Vitamins are organic compounds that assist in various bodily functions. For instance, Vitamin C supports the immune system, while Vitamin D aids in calcium absorption, essential for strong bones. Different vitamins have distinct roles, and a deficiency can lead to various health issues.

Minerals: Minerals are inorganic substances necessary for proper physiological functions. Calcium, for example, is vital for bone health, while iron is essential for oxygen transport in the blood. Minerals like potassium and magnesium are involved in maintaining proper muscle and nerve function.

The importance of macronutrients and micronutrients in nutrition lies in their ability to ensure that our bodies receive the necessary nutrients for growth, repair, and daily activities. A balanced diet that includes the right proportion of macronutrients and a variety of micronutrients is essential for overall health and well-being. It's not just about calories; it's about nourishing your body with the right combination of nutrients to thrive and lead a healthy life.

Story of Joe Cross:

Joe Cross is a prominent example of a person who underwent a remarkable transformation through the power of nutrition. In the documentary film "Fat, Sick & Nearly Dead," Joe shares his journey from being overweight, suffering from a debilitating autoimmune disease, and taking numerous medications to regain his health and vitality. Joe decided to embark on a 60-day juice fast, consuming only freshly extracted fruit and vegetable juices. This drastic change in his diet allowed him to flood his body with essential nutrients while eliminating processed foods and excessive calories. Over the course of those 60 days, he lost a significant amount of weight and saw a dramatic improvement in his health. Not only did Joe shed the excess pounds, but he was also able to reduce his reliance on medication, and eventually, he no longer needed them. His transformation inspired many others to take control of their health through nutrition and led to the creation of the "Reboot with Joe" community, which offers resources and support for people looking to make positive changes in their lives through juicing and healthy eating.

Joe Cross's story serves as a powerful testament to the potential of nutrition to transform one's life, both physically and mentally. It illustrates how making informed choices about what we eat can have a profound impact on our well-being. This is just one of many inspiring stories of individuals who have experienced life-changing transformations through nutrition. It highlights the importance of a balanced and healthy diet in achieving and maintaining good health.

Calories and Energy Balance: Explore the concept of calories and how they relate to energy balance, including the role of metabolism and weight management.

Calories and Energy Balance: What You Need to Know. Calories are like fuel for your body. Just like a car needs gas to run, your body needs calories to function. Here's how it works:

1. Calories In: When you eat or drink, you consume calories. These calories come from the foods and beverages you consume. Different foods have different calorie counts. For example, a salad might have fewer calories than a cheeseburger.

2. Calories Out: Your body burns calories throughout the day, even when you're resting.

Your basal metabolic rate (BMR) represents this concept. Beyond your BMR, engaging in physical activities such as walking or exercise also expends calories. The higher your activity level, the greater the calorie expenditure.

3. Achieving equilibrium: To maintain your weight, the calories you consume (calories in) should approximately match the calories you expend (calories out). This equilibrium is referred to as energy balance. If you ingest more calories than you utilize, weight gain follows. Conversely, a calorie deficit, where you burn more than you consume, leads to weight loss.

4. Weight management: If your goal is weight loss, generating a calorie deficit becomes imperative. This entails consuming fewer calories than you burn, attainable through portion control, selecting lower-calorie foods, and elevating physical activity.

5. Quality is crucial: Quantity isn't the sole factor; the nutritional value of your food holds significance as well. Prioritize nutrient-rich selections like fruits, vegetables, lean proteins, and whole grains, as they supply essential vitamins and minerals essential for your body's well-being.

Section 2: Understanding Dietary Patterns

Dietary Guidelines: Present the latest dietary guidelines and recommendations from health authorities to offer a framework for healthy eating. Dietary guidelines are like the road signs for a healthy lifestyle. They're practical tips and recommendations that help us make good choices about what we eat.

Here's a breakdown in a simple and understandable way:

1. Balanced Diet: whenever you want to eat puzzle, fill it with a mix of colorful fruits and vegetables, lean proteins like chicken or beans, whole grains like brown rice or whole wheat bread, and a dash of healthy fats like olive oil or nuts. This variety ensures you get all the nutrients your body needs.

2. Portion Control: Be mindful of your food intake, just as you carefully fill your car's gas tank without overflowing it. Embracing moderation when it comes to eating is key to sustaining a balanced and healthy weight.

3. Stay Hydrated: Just like a plant needs water to thrive, your body needs water to function properly. Drink plenty of water throughout the day.

4. Limit Sugar and Salt: Too much sugar and salt is like adding too much seasoning to your food. It can lead to health problems. Try to cut back on sugary drinks and snacks, and use herbs and spices to flavor your food instead of salt.

5. Choose Healthy Snacks: Snacking is okay, but choose wisely. Opt for fruits, veggies, or nuts as snacks instead of chips or candy.

6. Mindful Eating: Be mindful of your food choices and how they affect your body. Tune into your body's cues, eat until you're satisfied, and only when you're hungry.

7. Cook at Home: Cooking at home is like being the chef of your own restaurant. You have control over what goes into your meals, which can be healthier and more budget-friendly.

8. Limit Processed Foods: Consider processed foods as quick detours that may not be the healthiest choice. Aim to consume fresh, unprocessed foods whenever you can.

9. Enjoy Treats in Moderation: It's okay to enjoy your favorite treats occasionally, but don't make them a daily habit.

10. Be Patient: Just like a marathon, being healthy is a journey. Gradual alterations in your habits can ultimately result in significant enhancements to your well-being.

Cultural and Personal Influences: The tapestry of human existence is intricately woven with threads of cultural and personal influences, each contributing to the rich tapestry of our lives. These influences are the invisible hands that mold our beliefs, values, and worldviews, guiding us through the labyrinth of existence.

Cultural influences, like the vibrant colors of a mosaic, provide the backdrop against which our identities are forged. Our cultural heritage, language, traditions, and societal norms form the foundation upon which we build our sense of self. From the rhythm of our speech to the way we celebrate, our culture shapes the contours of our character.

Personal influences, on the other hand, are the unique brushstrokes on the canvas of our lives. They come from our individual experiences, relationships, and introspection. Our triumphs and tribulations, the people who have touched our hearts, and the choices we make all contribute to the masterpiece of our personal identity. Yet, these influences are not separate entities but rather intertwined in a dance of constant evolution. Our cultural background can profoundly impact our personal experiences, while our personal choices can redefine our cultural belonging. It is in this delicate interplay that we find the tapestry of our lives constantly shifting and reshaping. These influences are not passive forces; they hold the power to shape our perceptions, beliefs, and the way we engage with the world. They determine what we find meaningful, beautiful, or unsettling. They impact the way we communicate, empathize, and connect with others. Understanding the intricate web of cultural and personal influences is essential for self-discovery and fostering empathy towards others. It reminds us that our perspectives are but one facet of a multifaceted jewel, and that the beauty of humanity lies in its diversity.

"Cultural and Personal Influences" are the silent architects of our identities, the forces that shape the lens through which we view the world. They are a reminder that we are all products of our unique journeys, and that by appreciating the rich tapestry of influences in our lives, we can truly embrace the beauty of our shared human experience. Appreciate the impact of cultural heritage, individual tastes, and lifestyle decisions on shaping your dietary habits.

Section 3: Special Dietary Considerations

Diet and Disease: Examine the connection between diet and common health conditions like heart disease, diabetes, and obesity, emphasizing the role of preventive nutrition. Dietary Restrictions: Explore various dietary restrictions, such as vegetarianism, veganism, gluten-free diets, and food allergies, and provide guidance on meeting nutritional needs while adhering to these restrictions.

Section 4: Practical Tips and Strategies

Meal Planning: Offer practical tips for meal planning, including portion control, balanced meals, and mindful eating practices.

Label Reading: Teach readers how to decipher food labels and make informed choices at the grocery store.

Eating on a Budget: Share strategies for maintaining a healthy diet while managing budget constraints.

Section 5: Long-Term Health and Wellness

Sustainable Eating: Discuss the importance of sustainable food choices and their impact on both personal health and the environment. In a world where our choices have profound implications for the health of our planet, sustainable eating emerges as a powerful, conscientious solution. It's not just a trend; it's a fundamental shift in our approach to food that transcends the boundaries of culture, geography, and generations. Sustainable eating represents a harmonious relationship between our dietary habits and the Earth's fragile ecosystems, offering a unique and distinct path to a healthier, more equitable future.

At its core, sustainable eating is about redefining our connection with food. It challenges us to make choices that are not only good for our bodies but also for the environment. It's a departure from the era of convenience-driven, resource-intensive diets towards a mindset that honors the cycles of nature. By opting for locally sourced, seasonal produce, we reduce the carbon footprint of our meals, supporting local farmers and fostering a deeper connection to our surroundings.

One of the distinctive features of sustainable eating is its emphasis on biodiversity. While modern agriculture has, in many ways, simplified our food supply, it has also diminished genetic diversity and increased vulnerability to pests and diseases. Sustainable eating champions heirloom varieties and indigenous crops, celebrating the wealth of flavors, textures, and nutrients that nature offers. By doing so, it safeguards our food system against future uncertainties. sustainable eating encourages the responsible consumption of animal products. It advocates for reduced meat consumption and a shift towards ethically raised, pasture-fed livestock. This not only promotes animal welfare but also mitigates the environmental impact of industrial livestock farming, which is a leading contributor to deforestation, greenhouse gas emissions, and habitat loss.

In the context of sustainable eating, waste is seen as a resource to be minimized. Food scraps become compost, and leftovers are creatively transformed into new dishes. This mindful approach not only reduces landfill waste but also conserves resources that would otherwise be expended in the production of more food.

Sustainable eating extends its reach beyond our plates, engaging with broader ethical and social issues. It encourages fair labor practices in food production, striving to eliminate exploitation and injustice in the agricultural sector. By supporting fair trade and equitable food distribution, sustainable eating ensures that the benefits of a thriving food system are shared equitably among all stakeholders.

sustainable eating is a unique and distinct paradigm shift in the way we relate to food. It is a conscious choice to nourish ourselves in harmony with the planet. It celebrates the diversity of nature, respects the dignity of all living beings, and seeks to leave a bountiful legacy for future generations. By embracing sustainable eating, we not only satisfy our hunger but also feed the well-being of our planet.

Lifelong Habits: Encourage the development of lifelong healthy eating habits and provide strategies for maintaining a balanced diet over time.

As you dive into the pages of this chapter, remember that nutrition and diet are not just about counting calories but about nourishing your body for a vibrant, fulfilling life. Whether you're looking to improve your health, manage a specific condition, or simply want to make better food choices, the knowledge and insights within these pages will serve as your compass on the journey to a healthier, happier you.

This structured approach should help you build a comprehensive and engaging chapter on nutrition and diet for your book or project. Feel free to customize it further to suit your specific goals and audience.

Chapter 3

The Importance of Physical Activity

Physical activity is not merely a routine but a pivotal element in maintaining both physical and mental well-being. Its significance goes beyond the pursuit of an ideal body; it encompasses a holistic approach to a healthier life. Physical activity is a cornerstone of physical health. Regular exercise strengthens the cardiovascular system, improves bone density, and or simply want to make better food choices, the knowledge and insights within these pages will serve as your compass on the journey to a healthier, happier you.

This structured approach should help you build a comprehensive and engaging chapter on nutrition and diet for your book or project. Feel free to customize it further to suit your specific goals and audience.

Chapter 3

The Importance of Physical Activity

Physical activity is not merely a routine but a pivotal element in maintaining both physical and mental well-being. Its significance goes beyond the pursuit of an ideal body; it encompasses a holistic approach to a healthier life. Physical activity is a cornerstone of physical health. Regular exercise strengthens the cardiovascular system, improves bone density, and enhances muscle tone. It helps control weight, reducing the risk of obesity and related health issues. Additionally, physical activity boosts the immune system, making the body more resilient to infections.

Equally important is the impact on mental health. Engaging in physical activity releases endorphins, the body's natural mood lifters, reducing stress and anxiety. It fosters better sleep patterns, which in turn contributes to improved cognitive function and emotional stability. Physical activity can be a powerful tool in combating conditions like depression and ADHD.

The benefits extend to social aspects of life. Participation in team sports or group fitness activities fosters camaraderie and a sense of belonging. This can be instrumental in building social bonds and reducing feelings of isolation. Beyond individual well-being, physical activity plays a crucial role in community health. Promoting physical activity can reduce the burden on healthcare systems by preventing chronic diseases. It can also strengthen communities by providing opportunities for people to come together and share common interests. In essence, physical activity is not a mere option but a necessity for a fulfilling life. It impacts physical health, mental well-being, and social connections, making it an integral part of a vibrant and balanced existence. Embracing a lifestyle that prioritizes regular physical activity is an investment in one's present and future vitality.

Certainly, let's delve further into the importance of physical activity:

Enhanced Longevity: Regular physical activity is linked to a longer lifespan. Studies consistently show that individuals who engage in regular exercise tend to live longer and have a lower risk of premature death. In an era where scientific progress is rewriting the boundaries of what it means to be human, the concept of enhanced longevity stands at the forefront of our collective imagination. It's not merely about living longer; it's about unlocking the secrets of extended vitality and rewriting the narrative of aging itself.

Imagine a world where the sands of time are not a relentless adversary but a malleable resource. Enhanced longevity is not a mere desire for immortality, but a quest for a life that is not bound by the limitations of time, age, and disease. It's a journey into uncharted territory where science, technology, and human ambition converge. The foundation of enhanced longevity lies in the mastery of human biology. Researchers delve deep into the intricacies of cellular aging, seeking ways to slow down or even reverse the clock. Genetic engineering, regenerative medicine, and personalized treatments are at the vanguard of this revolution, promising to rejuvenate our bodies at the molecular level.

But enhanced longevity is not just a scientific endeavor; it's a societal transformation. It compels us to rethink the structure of our lives, from education and careers to relationships and retirement. It prompts us to redefine what it means to be young, middle-aged, or elderly. The boundaries between these stages blur, creating a tapestry of experiences that transcends generational norms.

Moreover, the ethical dimensions of enhanced longevity are profound. Who gets access to these life-extending technologies? How do we address issues of inequality and the potential for an ever-widening longevity gap between the privileged and the marginalized? These questions challenge us to navigate the moral complexities of this brave new world. Enhanced longevity isn't just about living longer; it's about living better. It's about savoring the full spectrum of human experiences, from the thrill of youthful discovery to the wisdom of age. It's about cherishing the moments with loved ones, pursuing passions, and contributing to society with a vigor that defies the calendar.

As we embark on this journey towards enhanced longevity, we stand at the threshold of a new era— one where the boundaries of human potential are redefined, and the very essence of what it means to be human evolves. It's a journey fraught with challenges and uncertainties, but it's also a testament to our indomitable spirit, our insatiable curiosity, and our unwavering belief in the limitless possibilities of tomorrow. Enhanced longevity is not just a quest for a longer life; it's a celebration of life itself.

Disease Prevention: Physical activity is a potent preventive measure against numerous chronic diseases. It reduces the risk of heart disease, stroke, two types of diabetes, certain are; cancer, and osteoporosis.

Physical activity is a powerful and essential tool in the prevention of various chronic diseases. Engaging in regular physical activity not only enhances one's overall well-being but also significantly reduces the risk of developing debilitating health conditions such as heart disease, stroke, type of diabetes; cancer, and osteoporosis. This chapter delves into the importance of physical activity as a preventive measure against these chronic diseases, shedding light on its mechanisms, recommended levels, and its wide-reaching benefits.

I. Preventing Heart Disease:

Heart disease, a leading cause of mortality worldwide, can be effectively prevented through physical activity. Regular exercise helps maintain a healthy weight, lowers blood pressure, and improves cholesterol levels. Additionally, physical activity promotes efficient blood circulation and reduces the risk of plaque buildup in arteries, mitigating the chances of heart attacks and other cardiovascular diseases.

II. Reducing the Risk of Stroke:

Physical activity plays a pivotal role in reducing the risk of stroke. Exercise helps control blood pressure, improves blood vessel function, and aids in weight management—all factors that contribute to a healthier circulatory system. By enhancing overall cardiovascular health, physical activity acts as a formidable defense against strokes.

III. Preventing Type 2 Diabetes:

Type of 2 diabetes is closely linked to lifestyle factors, including physical inactivity and obesity. Engaging in regular physical activity helps the body utilize insulin more effectively, thus regulating blood sugar levels. Moreover, exercise contributes to weight control and reduces visceral fat, lowering the risk of developing type 2 diabetes significantly.

IV. Guarding Against Certain Types of Cancer:

Physical activity has been associated with a decreased risk of various types of cancer, including colon, breast, and lung cancer. Regular exercise helps the body maintain a healthy weight and reduces inflammation, both of which are known risk factors for cancer development. Additionally, exercise may help regulate hormone levels, further reducing the likelihood of certain cancers.

V. Strengthening Bones and Preventing Osteoporosis:

Bones are the architectural framework of our bodies, providing structural support and protecting vital organs. Just like the foundation of a house, maintaining strong and healthy bones is crucial for a long and active life. Osteoporosis, a condition characterized by weakened and brittle bones, can have severe consequences, but it is preventable.

Osteoporosis is a condition characterized by fragile bones that are susceptible to fractures. Weight-bearing exercises, such as walking, jogging, and resistance training, stimulate bone formation and increase bone density. These activities play a crucial role in preventing osteoporosis and maintaining strong, healthy bones throughout life. Embracing physical activity as a lifelong commitment is a proactive step towards a healthier, disease-free future.

Improved Cognitive Function: Physical activity is not just beneficial for the body; it also nourishes the mind. Engaging in regular physical activity has been proven to be a transformative catalyst for your mind. It ignites cognitive faculties, strengthens memory retention, and sparks the fires of creativity. In essence, exercise is not just a workout for your body; it's a workout for your brain, propelling you toward sharper thinking and boundless imagination. It may even reduce the risk of cognitive decline as we age. Improved cognitive function need not follow a conventional path. By adopting a holistic approach that integrates mindfulness, nutrition, neurofeedback, creativity, and environmental optimization, individuals can unlock their cognitive potential in a unique and distinct way. This multifaceted approach empowers individuals to harness the power of their minds and embark on a journey of cognitive enhancement that goes beyond the ordinary In the pursuit of enhancing cognitive function, traditional approaches often prioritize the development of memory, attention, and problem-solving skills. While these methods undoubtedly hold value, a unique and distinct perspective on improving cognitive abilities involves a holistic approach that integrates mind, body, and environment. This write-up explores a multifaceted approach to achieving improved cognitive function that transcends the conventional.

Productivity and Focus: Engaging in physical activity can boost productivity and focus. Regular breaks for exercise during the workday can refresh the mind, leading to increased efficiency and creativity.

Healthy Aging: Physical activity is a key component of healthy aging. It helps maintain mobility and independence in older adults, reducing the risk of falls and injuries.

Stress Reduction: Exercise reduces the production of stress hormones and triggers the release of endorphins, promoting a sense of relaxation and well-being.

Positive Body Image: Regular physical activity encourages a positive body image by promoting self-confidence and self-esteem. It shifts the focus from appearance to what one's body can achieve.

Environmental Impact: Embracing active transportation options like walking or cycling reduces the carbon footprint, contributing to a cleaner and more sustainable environment.

Role Modeling: Engaging in physical activity sets a positive example for others, especially children. It encourages them to adopt healthy habits from a young age.

Quality of Life: Ultimately, physical activity enhances the overall quality of life. It provides a sense of accomplishment, happiness, and a feeling of vitality that permeates all aspects of daily living. In a world increasingly dominated by sedentary lifestyles, recognizing the multifaceted importance of physical activity becomes imperative. It's not just about looking good; it's about feeling good, being healthy, and living life to its fullest potential. Integrating regular exercise into our lives is an investment that pays dividends in health, happiness, and longevity.

Chapter 4

Sleep and Its Role in Holistic Health

Sleep is not merely a nightly ritual; it's a cornerstone of holistic health, fostering vitality in mind, body, and spirit. In a world perpetually in motion, the profound influence of sleep often goes overlooked, but its significance cannot be overstated. Physiologically, sleep is a complex dance of restoration. During the night, the body repairs tissues, consolidates memories, and regulates hormones, contributing to a robust immune system and optimal metabolic function. It's a time when the brain meticulously files away information, clearing the mental clutter and preparing us for another day of learning and growth. Beyond its physiological prowess, sleep transcends into the realm of emotional well-being. It is the balm for emotional wounds, a source of resilience, and a guardian against mood disorders. Inadequate sleep can lead to heightened stress levels, anxiety, and even depression, emphasizing its indispensable role in nurturing mental equilibrium.

The relationship between sleep and physical health is irrefutable. Chronic sleep deprivation is associated with an increased risk of cardiovascular diseases, diabetes, obesity, and compromised immune responses. In contrast, prioritizing quality sleep can be a formidable shield against these maladies, empowering the body to flourish in a state of equilibrium.

But sleep's holistic influence extends even further. It fosters creativity, enhances problem-solving abilities, and stimulates innovation. A well-rested mind is more adaptable and resilient, ready to embrace life's challenges with clarity and vigor.

In the pursuit of holistic health, sleep is the quiet hero that binds the various facets of our well-being. It fortifies the body's defenses, calms the turbulent seas of the mind, and nourishes the spirit. It's a pillar upon which our vitality stands, a bridge between the past and future, and a sanctuary where healing and renewal flourish.

To truly embrace holistic health, one must not underestimate the power of sleep. It's a unique and distinct ally, offering a wealth of benefits to those who honor its importance. So, when the night falls and the world quiets down, remember that sleep is not just a luxury; it's a precious investment in your holistic well-being.

Let's delve deeper into the role of sleep in holistic health:

Physical Restoration: Sleep is the body's natural reset button. During deep sleep stages, tissues are repaired, and muscle growth occurs. The immune system also gets a boost, helping the body defend against illness and disease. Furthermore, hormones like growth hormone and insulin are regulated during sleep, contributing to overall physical health. Physical restoration through sleep is an indispensable facet of our well-being, an intricate process where our bodies embark on a remarkable journey towards rejuvenation and recovery. This nightly odyssey, often underestimated in its significance, is an exquisite dance of biology and physiology.

During the initial stages of sleep, our bodies descend into a state of relaxation. Muscles relax, heart rate decelerates, and blood pressure gradually declines. This tranquil phase is essential for reducing the wear and tear that our bodies endure throughout the day. It's a moment of respite for our weary limbs and overworked organs. As we venture deeper into slumber, the magic unfolds. Our cells become diligent workers, repairing damaged tissues and fortifying our immune system. The brain, the orchestrator of this symphony, orchestrates the release of growth hormones, fostering the renewal of skin, bone, and muscle. Collagen production spikes, contributing to skin's elasticity and vitality. Even our precious memories are safeguarded and consolidated during this nocturnal voyage. Perhaps the most profound act of restoration transpires in the brain. It's a cerebral cleansing of sorts, where toxins and waste products are expelled through the glymphatic system, making way for cognitive clarity upon awakening. Neuronal connections are strengthened, creativity is nurtured, and emotional equilibrium is restored. Physical restoration during sleep is like nature's gift to our bodies, a silent remedy for the bruises and stresses of life. It's an intricate choreography where each part of our being plays a role, weaving a tapestry of renewal. To disregard the importance of sleep is to undermine our body's innate wisdom, for it is in the embrace of slumber that we find the physical restoration that is essential for our continued vitality and well-being.

Cognitive Function: Sleep serves as a beneficial role in cognitive function. It's during deep sleep that the brain consolidates memories, allowing us to retain information and learn effectively. Sleep also clears out toxins that accumulate during wakefulness, promoting optimal brain function. In the intricate symphony of our mental processes, sleep serves as the conductor, orchestrating a mesmerizing performance of cognitive function. Deep sleep, the maestro of this nocturnal masterpiece, takes center stage, weaving together the threads of memory. It's in the velvety embrace of deep slumber that our brains delicately stitch the tapestry of experiences, transforming them into lasting memories.

But sleep's role transcends the boundaries of memory alone; it transcends into the realm of purification. In the hushed moments of night, as our consciousness retreats, sleep becomes the custodian of a unique cleansing ritual. It sweeps away the clutter and detritus of our waking hours, the metabolic waste and toxins that accumulate during our journey through the day. In doing so, sleep offers a fresh canvas to our brain, a pristine stage for the next day's cognitive performance. In essence, sleep isn't just a passive interlude between waking hours; it is an active curator of our cognitive prowess. It is the custodian of our memories and the purifier of our mental sanctum. It orchestrates the harmony of our thoughts, allowing us to learn, adapt, and thrive in the ever-evolving theater of life."

Emotional Well-Being: A good night's sleep can help regulate mood, reduce stress, and enhance emotional resilience. On the flip side, chronic sleep deprivation can lead to mood disorders like depression and anxiety. Emotional well-being is intricately intertwined with the quality of our sleep, forming a delicate balance that profoundly influences our mental state. Imagine sleep as the master conductor of an orchestra, where each note represents an emotion. A harmonious night's rest orchestrates a symphony of positive emotions, allowing them to resonate with clarity and precision. When we experience a good night's sleep, the conductor skillfully navigates through the emotional repertoire. It fine-tunes our mood, tempering any dissonance, and fortifying the crescendo of contentment. Stress, akin to a discordant note, is skillfully subdued, and emotional resilience takes center stage, enhancing our ability to confront life's challenges with poise.

However, when the conductor is deprived of the necessary hours and consistency, the emotional symphony becomes chaotic. Chronic sleep deprivation disrupts the rhythm, leading to a cacophony of negative emotions. Depression and anxiety, like unruly soloists, seize the spotlight. Their solos overpower the harmonious melodies of happiness and serenity. A restful night's sleep composes a sonata of emotional balance, while sleep deprivation orchestrates a dissonant composition of mood disorders. Recognizing this intricate connection reminds us of the pivotal role sleep plays in nurturing our emotional well-being.

Physical Health: Lack of sleep has been linked to an increased risk of various health problems, including cardiovascular diseases, diabetes, and obesity. Sleep influences appetite-regulating hormones, which can lead to overeating and weight gain when sleep is insufficient. In the intricate symphony of our well-being, sleep plays the role of a silent conductor, directing the harmonious functioning of our physical health. Its absence, like a discordant note, can trigger a cascade of consequences that resonate throughout our body.

Consider the delicate balance of cardiovascular health. Sleep is not merely a pause in our daily rhythm but a crucial maintenance period for our heart and blood vessels. When this nocturnal restoration is disrupted, the risk of cardiovascular diseases rises, akin to a disrupted melody in an orchestra.

Sleep, it seems, also dabbles in the realm of metabolism. It possesses a unique power to sway our appetite-regulating hormones, like a maestro guiding the tempo of a composition. Inadequate sleep can send these hormones into disarray, leading to an increased appetite and, ultimately, a crescendo of overeating and weight gain. So, let us cherish our nights of slumber, for they are not just mere respites from the day's hustle and bustle. They are the orchestrators of our physical well-being, the conductors of our health symphony, and the guardians of a harmonious existence."

Mental Clarity: Slumber revitalizes the intellect, paving the way for heightened concentration, effective troubleshooting, and innovative thinking. When well-rested, individuals tend to make better decisions and are more innovative in their thinking.

Imagine your mind as a vast landscape, constantly traversed by thoughts, ideas, and emotions. Mental clarity is like the clear blue sky above this landscape, offering an unobstructed view of your inner world. Sleep serves as the dedicated gardener of this landscape, tirelessly tending to the garden of your thoughts. During sleep, your brain engages in a meticulous pruning process, trimming away the excess mental foliage that has accumulated during the day. This pruning not only removes clutter but also allows the most important ideas and memories to flourish, much like a skilled bonsai artist shaping a miniature tree. As dawn breaks and you awaken from a restful night's sleep, your mental garden is resplendent, with vibrant, well-nurtured thoughts and ideas. This rejuvenation isn't merely about feeling well-rested; it's about the profound impact on your cognitive abilities. With a clear mental canvas, you're better equipped to focus on tasks, as if a spotlight shines directly on the matter at hand. Problem-solving becomes a seamless journey through your well-organized mental pathways, and creativity blossoms as your mind is free to explore uncharted territories without the weeds of fatigue and mental fog hindering your way.

Furthermore, well-rested individuals are akin to skilled navigators, making precise decisions with clarity and conviction. They can chart new courses, unafraid of venturing into the unknown, because they know their mental compass is finely tuned. Mental clarity, cultivated through the nurturing embrace of sleep, allows you to explore the uncharted depths of your own creativity and intellect, making it a cornerstone for better decision-making and innovative thinking. Just as a garden thrives with proper care, so does the mind when granted the gift of restorative sleep.

Stress Reduction: Sleep acts as a buffer against stress. It provides a crucial period for the body to recover from the physical and emotional demands of the day. A good night's sleep can make challenging situations feel more manageable.

"Envision sleep as the uncelebrated champion of your everyday existence, silently weaving its enchantment during your repose.

In the realm of stress management, sleep stands as a formidable shield. It's your body's way of saying, 'Let's hit the reset button.' When you lay down to rest, your physical and emotional batteries recharge, ready to face another day.

Consider it a sanctuary for your mind and body, where the chaos of daily life subsides, and tranquility takes over. In the cocoon of a good night's sleep, your brain sifts through the experiences of the day, processing emotions, and weaving them into a coherent narrative. This process, almost like a nightly therapy session, helps you wake up feeling more emotionally resilient and prepared for whatever challenges may lie ahead.

Moreover, sleep has this remarkable ability to transform daunting obstacles into manageable hurdles. Imagine a day filled with demands, deadlines, and decisions that seem insurmountable. After a night of restorative sleep, those same challenges don't appear as menacing. You wake up with a newfound clarity and perspective, ready to tackle whatever life throws your way. So, in the grand tapestry of self-care, don't underestimate the role of sleep. It's not just about resting; it's about fortifying your mind, body, and spirit against the storms of daily life. Embrace the power of sleep, and you'll find that even the most daunting days can be conquered with grace and resilience."

Holistic Balance: Holistic well-being entails considering the entirety of an individual, encompassing their mental, physical, and spiritual dimensions.

When you prioritize sleep, you're investing in your overall well-being, achieving balance in your life. Holistic health is an approach that considers the entire person, recognizing that our well-being is not just physical but also involves mental, emotional, and spiritual aspects. It emphasizes that these aspects are interconnected and should be addressed together to achieve true health.

Sleep is the foundation upon which holistic health is built. It's the bridge between our physical, mental, and emotional well-being. Neglecting sleep can lead to a breakdown in these interconnected systems, whereas valuing and nurturing it empowers us to lead healthier, more fulfilling lives. It's a unique and distinct contributor to holistic health, one that should not be underestimated or sacrificed in the hustle and bustle of modern life.

Chapter 5

Holistic Approaches to Preventative Healthcare

In an era where healthcare is a paramount concern for individuals and societies alike, a holistic approach to preventative healthcare emerges as a beacon of hope. This distinctive approach transcends the conventional model of treating symptoms and delves deeper into the realms of overall well-being. By addressing the physical, mental, emotional, and even spiritual aspects of health, holistic preventative healthcare seeks to empower individuals to take charge of their own wellness journey. At the core of holistic preventative healthcare is the understanding that health is not merely the absence of disease but a dynamic balance between mind, body, and spirit. It emphasizes the importance of proactive measures to maintain this equilibrium.

Picture your health as a puzzle with many pieces: your body, your mind, your emotions, and even your spirit. Holistic preventative healthcare is like putting together this puzzle to keep you healthy and happy.

Let's break it down in a simple, practical way:

1. Mind Your Mind: Your thoughts and feelings impact your health. Take a few minutes each day to clear your mind through activities like deep breathing, meditation, or just a peaceful walk. Less stress means better health.

 "Mind Your Mind," let's explore the profound connection between your inner world and your overall well-being. Your thoughts and emotions wield a subtle yet potent influence on your physical health, making it imperative to cultivate a harmonious mental landscape. Imagine your mind as a serene garden, where each thought and emotion is a blooming flower. By dedicating a few precious minutes daily, you embark on a journey of tending to this garden. Through the gentle practice of deep breathing, you not only oxygenate your body but also nurture the soil of your consciousness. Meditation, a gateway to tranquility, allows you to prune away the weeds of anxiety and cultivate the lushness of inner peace. Moreover, consider the simple act of a peaceful walk, where your every step resonates with mindfulness. As your feet connect with the earth, your mind synchronizes with the rhythm of nature, unfurling the canvas of serenity. In these moments, you become the artist, painting your mental landscape with the soothing hues of calmness.

Why is all this important? Because the tapestry of your mental state profoundly influences your health. Stress, like a relentless storm, can erode the foundations of well-being. Conversely, by tending to your inner garden, you fortify your mental resilience, erecting a barrier against the tempests of stress. This, in turn, paves the way for the flourishing of better health.

So, remember, "Mind Your Mind" isn't just a phrase; it's a profound invitation to cultivate a sanctuary of serenity within yourself, where the blossoms of tranquility yield the fruits of vitality.

2. Eat Real Food: Forget diets; focus on real, unprocessed foods. Load your dish with a vibrant array of fruits and vegetables, along with lean protein sources and whole grains. This ensures your body receives the optimal sustenance to maintain its vigor.

In today's fast-paced world, where fad diets and quick fixes dominate the health and wellness landscape, the timeless advice to "Eat Real Food" stands out as a beacon of sensible and sustainable nutrition. This simple yet profound mantra emphasizes the importance of prioritizing whole, unprocessed foods over artificial or highly processed alternatives.

First and foremost, the phrase encourages us to forget about diets. Diets often come and go, promising rapid weight loss or other health benefits but frequently fail to deliver long-term results. Instead of hopping from one diet trend to another, the focus shifts to a more fundamental and enduring approach: nourishing your body with real, wholesome foods. The heart of the "Eat Real Food" philosophy lies in the composition of your plate. When you fill it with colorful fruits and vegetables, you are not just adding vibrant flavors and textures to your meals; you are also providing your body with a rich array of essential vitamins, minerals, and antioxidants. These nutrients are critical for overall health, immune function, and disease prevention. The variety of colors on your plate represents a diverse range of nutrients, ensuring that your body gets what it needs. Lean proteins are another cornerstone of this approach. Including sources like poultry, fish, tofu, legumes, and lean cuts of meat provides your body with essential amino acids necessary for muscle repair and growth. Proteins also help you feel fuller for longer, reducing the likelihood of unhealthy snacking and overeating.

Whole grains complete the trifecta of real food. Foods like brown rice, quinoa, and whole wheat bread are rich in fiber, which aids digestion, stabilizes blood sugar levels, and helps maintain a healthy weight. Unlike their refined counterparts, whole grains retain the bran and germ, ensuring that you benefit from the full spectrum of nutrients. By adhering to the "Eat Real Food" mantra, you're not just making a dietary choice; you're making a lifestyle choice. This approach transcends temporary food restrictions and encourages a more holistic perspective on nutrition. It's about fostering a relationship with food that promotes well-being, sustains energy levels, and supports longevity.

Furthermore, this philosophy aligns with the idea that food is not merely fuel; it's a form of self-care. By choosing real, unprocessed foods, you're showing yourself the respect and care you deserve. This mindset shift can lead to greater mindfulness in your eating habits, helping you make choices that benefit your long-term health.

"Eat Real Food" is a powerful reminder to prioritize quality and nutrition over quick fixes and restrictive diets. It encourages the consumption of colorful fruits and vegetables, lean proteins, and whole grains as the foundation of a healthy diet. This approach is not just about what you eat; it's about how you approach food and nutrition as a whole, promoting a sustainable and nourishing relationship with what you put on your plate.

3. Keep Moving: You don't need to be a gym enthusiast. Find an activity you enjoy, whether it's dancing, walking, or playing a sport. Moving regularly helps keep your body in good shape. You don't have to transform into a fitness fanatic to ensure your physical well-being. Instead, discover an activity that genuinely excites you, be it dancing, strolling through the park, or engaging in a favorite sport. Engaging in regular physical activity offers a multitude of benefits that go far beyond just aesthetics; it's about nurturing your overall health and well-being.

One of the key advantages of staying active is the positive impact it has on your physical health. It promotes cardiovascular health by strengthening your heart and improving blood circulation. Regular movement also helps in maintaining a healthy weight, reducing the risk of obesity and related health issues such as diabetes and joint problems. Moreover, it enhances muscle tone and flexibility, contributing to a better posture and reducing the chances of muscle-related injuries. Not only does physical activity fortify the body, but it also has a profound effect on mental health. Engaging in activities you love can release endorphins, those wonderful 'feel-good' hormones that boost your mood and alleviate stress and anxiety. It can be a potent tool in managing mental health conditions like depression.

In addition to the physical and mental benefits, staying active can be a social experience. Joining a dance class, walking group, or sports team provides an opportunity to connect with others who share similar interests, fostering a sense of community and friendship. This social aspect of physical activity can be equally vital for mental and emotional well-being. Making movement a regular part of your life can increase your overall energy levels. You'll find yourself feeling more vibrant and alert, which can improve productivity in everyday tasks and work. It can also lead to better sleep patterns, as physical activity often results in a more restful night's sleep. The beauty of staying active is that there's no one-size-fits-all approach. The key is to find what sparks your passion and keeps you motivated. It might be a solo endeavor like morning yoga, or a team sport like soccer. Experiment, explore, and embrace the joy of moving your body in ways that bring you happiness.

'Keep Moving' is not just a piece of advice; it's a mantra for a healthier, happier life. Regardless of your fitness level, incorporating regular physical activity into your routine is a gift you give to yourself. It's a journey towards improved physical and mental health, enhanced social connections, heightened energy levels, and a brighter outlook on life. So, find your movement, keep it enjoyable, and relish the journey towards a healthier you."

4. Try Alternative Therapies: Don't shy away from things like acupuncture, massage, or herbal remedies if they interest you. These can complement traditional medicine and make you feel better.

• Acupuncture: Acupuncture, an age-old Chinese tradition, encompasses the insertion of slender needles into precise locations on the body to ignite the flow of vital energy. Proponents believe it can help alleviate a variety of health issues, including pain, stress, and digestive problems. While scientific research is ongoing, many individuals report experiencing relief and improved vitality through acupuncture sessions. It's important to consult a licensed acupuncturist for safe and effective treatment.

- **Massage Therapy:** Massage therapy is a well-known method for promoting relaxation and reducing muscle tension. Beyond its soothing effects, it can aid in relieving pain and improving circulation. Various massage techniques, such as Swedish, deep tissue, and hot stone massage, cater to different needs. Regular massages can contribute to reduced stress levels and an enhanced sense of well-being.

- **Herbal Remedies:** Herbal remedies involve using plant-based substances to address various health concerns. These remedies have been employed for centuries across different cultures. For instance, herbs like ginger and chamomile are known for their digestive benefits, while others like echinacea are used to boost the immune system. Incorporating herbal teas, supplements, or tinctures into your routine can provide natural support for specific health goals. However, it's essential to consult with an herbalist or healthcare professional to ensure safety and efficacy.

It's important to remember that while alternative therapies can be beneficial, they are not a replacement for medical advice or treatment when needed. It's wise to consult with healthcare professionals who can help you create a well-rounded healthcare plan that may include both traditional medicine and alternative therapies to optimize your health and well-being. Always ensure that any practitioners you work with are qualified and experienced in their respective fields.

5. Talk It Out: Your emotional well-being matters.Open up about your emotions to friends, family members, or seek support from a professional counselor. Keeping emotions bottled up can harm your health. It's not just a matter of feeling good; it's about ensuring that your body and mind function optimally. One of the most effective ways to safeguard your emotional well-being is by engaging in open and honest communication. In the hustle and bustle of our modern lives, we often find ourselves juggling numerous responsibilities, from work demands to family obligations. It's easy to let our emotions take a backseat amidst this chaos, but doing so can have severe consequences for our physical and mental health.

Imagine your emotions as a pressure cooker. When you keep them bottled up, the pressure builds, and eventually, it's bound to explode. This explosion can manifest in various ways, such as anxiety, depression, or even physical health issues like high blood pressure or chronic pain. So, addressing your emotions is not just a matter of convenience; it's a necessity. Sharing your feelings with others is like releasing the valve on that emotional pressure cooker. Whether it's with a close friend, a family member, or a professional counselor, talking about what's on your mind can provide profound relief. It's a way to process your thoughts and feelings, gain new perspectives, and, most importantly, feel heard and understood. In these chapter, you're not burdening others with your problems; you're sharing a part of yourself and creating a bond of trust and support. It's a reciprocal process; just as you confide in others, they can do the same with you. This exchange of emotions fosters stronger connections and deeper relationships. Speaking with a counselor or therapist offers a structured and confidential environment where you can explore your emotions and develop coping strategies. They are trained to provide guidance and tools to help you navigate life's challenges.

So, remember, when you "Talk It Out," you're not just safeguarding your emotional well-being; you're investing in your overall health. It's a proactive step towards leading a balanced, fulfilling life, free from the detrimental effects of bottled-up emotions."

6. Connect and Find Purpose: Building strong relationships and finding meaning in life is good for your soul and health. Spend time with loved ones and explore what makes you happy.

Connection and Relationships:

Human beings are inherently social creatures. Our ability to form connections and relationships with others is a fundamental aspect of our nature. These connections go beyond mere social interactions; they are the building blocks of emotional support systems that sustain us through life's challenges. When we spend time with loved ones, we cultivate a sense of belonging and connectedness. These connections provide a support network that bolsters our mental and emotional well-being. Whether it's family, friends, or a significant other, these relationships offer comfort, reassurance, and a sense of security. Strong relationships also contribute to lower stress levels. When we have people we can confide in and lean on during difficult times, the body releases fewer stress hormones. This reduction in stress has a cascade of positive effects on our overall health, from improving heart health to boosting our immune system.

Finding Purpose and Meaning:

Beyond relationships, finding purpose and meaning in life is a profound pursuit. It's about discovering what truly matters to you and aligning your actions with those values. This pursuit often involves introspection and self-discovery. When you find your purpose, life takes on new meaning. You wake up each day with a sense of direction and motivation. This sense of purpose not only enhances your psychological well-being but also influences your physical health. People who live purposeful lives tend to make healthier choices, such as exercising regularly and maintaining a balanced diet. In the midst of challenges, having a sense of purpose acts as a wellspring of resilience. When you have a clear sense of why you're here and what you're working towards, it becomes easier to navigate life's challenges. This resilience can positively affect everything from mental health to longevity.

The Interplay:

The beautiful interplay between strong relationships and a sense of purpose becomes evident when you consider that these two elements often complement each other. Meaningful relationships can help you discover your purpose by exposing you to different perspectives and opportunities. Conversely, a clear sense of purpose can enhance your relationships, as it allows you to bring more authenticity and intention into your interactions. Connecting with loved ones and finding purpose in life are not just abstract concepts; they are essential aspects of holistic well-being. They nurture your soul, reduce stress, improve mental health, and even have a positive impact on your physical health. In the intricate tapestry of life, these elements are the threads that create a vibrant and fulfilling existence.

7. Check Your Health: Regular check-ups are like car maintenance; they catch problems early. Don't skip them, but remember that staying healthy isn't just about doctor visits.

Imagine your body as a finely tuned machine, much like a high-performance car. Just as you wouldn't neglect routine maintenance for your prized vehicle, you shouldn't skip regular health check-ups for your most valuable asset – your health. These health check-ups serve as the diagnostic tools of your well-being, designed not only to catch problems early but also to fine-tune and optimize your body's functioning. Much like a skilled mechanic identifies issues in your car's engine before they become major breakdowns, your doctor can detect health concerns before they escalate into serious illnesses. But here's the twist: maintaining your health isn't solely reliant on these check-ups. While they are crucial, a truly holistic approach to well-being goes beyond the confines of a doctor's office. It's about recognizing that staying healthy is a lifestyle, not a once-a-year event.

In this journey toward well-being, diet, exercise, stress management, and mental health play pivotal roles. Think of them as the high-octane fuel, regular maintenance, and state-of-the-art technology that your body needs to perform at its best. Just as a sports car demands the right fuel and diligent care to deliver peak performance, your body thrives when nourished, exercised, and nurtured with mindfulness. So, yes, regular health check-ups are indispensable. They are the pit stops where you assess your progress and address any underlying issues. But they are just one part of the equation. True health, like a high-performance car, is a harmonious blend of meticulous care, proactive maintenance, and the drive to continually improve.

View your health as a masterpiece that requires meticulous attention, much like a luxury car. Embrace regular check-ups as a part of this process, but also remember that your daily habits and choices are the fuel that propels you toward a healthier, more vibrant life.

8. Make Small Changes: Big changes are hard, so start small. Maybe swap a sugary drink for water, take a short walk daily, or set aside time to relax. Small steps add up to big improvements. self-improvement and personal development, the idea of "making small changes" is akin to the subtle yet powerful strokes of a skilled artist. Imagine you're standing in front of a blank canvas, representing your life, and you have a vision of a magnificent masterpiece you want to create. It's vast, intricate, and seems overwhelming at first glance. However, you understand that every masterpiece begins with a single brushstroke, a solitary note, or a lone word.

Thus, making small changes becomes your artistic approach to life's canvas. You recognize that big changes can be daunting and often unsustainable. They require immense energy, commitment, and sometimes, they trigger resistance. But, by starting small, you're implementing a strategy that is not only manageable but also psychologically astute.

Let's delve into some practical examples:

Swap Sugary Drinks for Water: Imagine this as selecting the perfect color palette for your artwork. Instead of abruptly eliminating all sugary drinks, you decide to start by replacing just one daily soda with a refreshing glass of water. This small shift might seem inconsequential initially, but it's the foundation of a healthier lifestyle. Over time, as you enjoy the benefits of increased hydration and reduced sugar intake, you'll be inspired to make more mindful choices about what you consume.

Take a Short Walk Daily: Think of this as adding delicate brushstrokes to your canvas. Instead of committing to a grueling exercise regimen that you might dread, you choose to take a short walk every day. This gentle movement not only promotes physical well-being but also provides you with precious moments of solitude and reflection. As you step outside and breathe in the fresh air, you'll gradually find yourself craving longer walks, exploring new paths, and embracing a more active lifestyle.

Set Aside Time to Relax: This is like choosing the perfect background for your artwork. In the chaos of daily life, carving out even a few minutes of relaxation can feel like a luxury. However, by dedicating a small portion of your day to unwind, whether it's through meditation, reading, or simply enjoying a cup of tea, you're laying the groundwork for reduced stress and increased mental clarity. These moments of reprieve will accumulate, allowing you to approach challenges with a greater sense of calm and creativity. The beauty of this approach lies in its cumulative effect. Like an artist who patiently layers colors and textures to create a masterpiece, you're building a life of purpose and fulfillment one small change at a time. Each brushstroke, each step, and each moment of relaxation adds depth and richness to your canvas, gradually transforming it into the masterpiece you envisioned. So, remember, when faced with the daunting prospect of change, think small. Embrace the power of incremental progress, and you'll find that these seemingly insignificant shifts are the threads that weave the fabric of your personal growth and transformation. Over time, the big changes you once feared will emerge naturally and effortlessly, seamlessly integrated into the beautiful tapestry of your life.

Holistic healthcare is about putting all these pieces together. When you do, you'll have a complete picture of your health and can take steps to prevent problems. It's like taking care of your body, mind, and soul, all rolled into one. Simple, right?

Chapter 6

Spirituality and Its Influence on Well-Being

In the tapestry of human existence, spirituality is a thread that weaves through the very essence of our being. It transcends the boundaries of religious dogma and ritual, touching the core of our existence. This chapter embarks on an exploration of spirituality's multifaceted influence on well-being, delving into the profound ways it shapes our mental, emotional, and physical states.

Defining Spirituality:

Spirituality, a concept both nebulous and deeply personal, defies precise definition. It is the intimate journey to connect with something greater than ourselves, be it a higher power, the cosmos, or simply the profound mysteries of life. While spirituality often intersects with religion, it is not confined by it, encompassing a vast spectrum of beliefs and practices. Spirituality is a concept that dances on the edges of definition, ever-elusive and profoundly personal. It is the quest for a connection that transcends the boundaries of the self, a journey that beckons us to explore realms beyond the tangible. At its core, spirituality is the art of forging a profound link with something greater than ourselves, whether we envision this as a divine presence, the expansive cosmos, or the enigmatic tapestry of existence. What sets spirituality apart is its innate freedom, an emancipation from the rigid structures of organized religion. While it often weaves its threads into the fabric of faith and religious traditions, spirituality knows no confinement to dogma or creed. Instead, it sprawls across a vast spectrum of beliefs, embracing an inclusivity that welcomes seekers of all backgrounds and persuasions. In the realm of spirituality, one may find solace in the quiet contemplation of nature's wonders, seeking divinity in the rustling leaves of a forest or the shimmering stars of a night sky. Others may embark on an inner odyssey through meditation, delving deep into the recesses of the mind to discover the whispers of their own souls. For some, spirituality unfolds in acts of compassion and selflessness, as they strive to be vessels of love and kindness in a world often marred by discord. This mystical journey may be solitary or shared, guided by ancient wisdom or personal revelation. It invites us to question, explore, and transcend the boundaries of our physical existence. Spirituality is, in its essence, an unwavering pursuit of meaning, an acknowledgment that there is more to life than what meets the eye.

So, while the definition of spirituality remains elusive, its essence remains a beacon of hope and understanding in an ever-changing world. It reminds us that, in the vast tapestry of human experience, there is room for the pursuit of the ineffable, the quest for the sublime, and the unending exploration of the mysteries that surround us."

Spirituality and Emotional Well-Being:

Balancing emotional well-being involves a graceful interplay of comprehending, handling, and articulating our emotions. In its diverse manifestations, spirituality offers a valuable component in this equation. Spirituality, in its various forms, provides a nurturing space for this dance. It offers solace through meditation, prayer, or contemplation, enabling individuals to find refuge amidst the turbulence of their emotions. Furthermore, it fosters empathy, compassion, and a sense of interconnectedness, which in turn promotes emotional resilience.

• Spirituality and Mental Well-Being:

The human mind is a vast landscape of thoughts, beliefs, and perceptions. Spirituality can be a compass guiding this inner terrain. Practices such as mindfulness and self-reflection, often intertwined with spirituality, cultivate mental clarity and equanimity. Moreover, belief systems that emphasize purpose and meaning can serve as powerful buffers against existential angst and depression. The human mind, an intricate mosaic of thoughts and emotions, constantly seeks equilibrium. In this perpetual journey towards mental well-being, spirituality emerges as an invaluable compass. It is within this intricate relationship that we explore how spirituality, mindfulness, self-reflection, and a sense of purpose converge to create a distinct path towards enhancing mental clarity, equanimity, and resilience. Mindfulness, a practice deeply rooted in spirituality, encourages individuals to anchor themselves in the present moment. By focusing on their breath, sensations, or surroundings, individuals can detach from the whirlwind of thoughts that often engulfs the mind. This practice allows one to observe thoughts without judgment, fostering self-awareness and acceptance. In doing so, mindfulness becomes a powerful tool for cultivating mental clarity. It encourages individuals to see their thoughts as passing clouds, not absolute truths, thereby diminishing the power of negative or distressing thinking patterns.

Simultaneously, spirituality and self-reflection are intertwined processes that promote mental well-being. Self-reflection involves an introspective journey, a conscious effort to understand one's beliefs, values, and experiences. In this endeavor, spirituality offers a unique framework for exploring the self. It encourages individuals to delve into profound questions about their existence, purpose, and connection to the universe. Self-reflection within a spiritual context can uncover deeper layers of understanding, leading to personal growth and emotional healing. It provides a space for individuals to reconcile their inner conflicts and gain clarity about their values, thus contributing to a more stable and balanced mental state. However, the most profound impact of spirituality on mental well-being may arise from belief systems that emphasize purpose and meaning. Humans are inherently driven by a quest for meaning in their lives. Spirituality often offers a rich tapestry of narratives and philosophies that provide answers to existential questions. Whether through organized religion, philosophy, or individual spiritual practices, belief in a higher purpose can be a formidable buffer against existential angst and depression. When individuals find meaning in their experiences and a sense of connection to something greater than themselves, they become more resilient in the face of life's challenges. The interplay between spirituality, mindfulness, self-reflection, and purpose forms a unique and distinct path towards enhancing mental well-being. This path invites individuals to explore the depths of their inner world, fostering self-awareness, resilience, and emotional equilibrium. It reminds us that, in the vast landscape of the human mind, spirituality can serve as a guiding light, illuminating the path towards mental clarity, equanimity, and purposeful living.

- Spirituality and Physical Well-Being:

The mind and body are not distinct entities but intricately linked. Spirituality recognizes this symbiosis and acknowledges the impact of our mental and emotional states on physical health. Studies have shown that practices like meditation and yoga, rooted in spirituality, reduce stress, lower blood pressure, and enhance overall physical well-being. Furthermore, the sense of purpose derived from spiritual beliefs can stimulate the body's natural healing processes.

The intricate dance between our mental and physical well-being is a phenomenon often overlooked in our fast-paced lives. However, spirituality, with its unique lens, sheds light on this interconnectedness, offering a profound perspective on the union of the mind and body.

At its core, spirituality posits that the mind and body are not distinct entities but rather intimately intertwined. It acknowledges the profound influence of our mental and emotional states on our physical health. This perspective heralds a paradigm shift, emphasizing that achieving physical well-being necessitates nurturing our mental and emotional states.

Numerous scientific studies have illuminated the tangible benefits of incorporating spiritual practices into our lives. Meditation and yoga, deeply rooted in spiritual traditions, have garnered attention for their remarkable impact on health. These practices act as bridges, uniting the ethereal realm of the mind with the corporeal realm of the body. Meditation, for instance, has been scientifically proven to reduce stress levels. In the hustle and bustle of modern life, stress is a ubiquitous companion, wreaking havoc on our bodies. Yet, when we embark on a spiritual journey through meditation, we unlock the power to soothe our minds, and in turn, our bodies. The deep relaxation and mindfulness cultivated in meditation initiate a cascade of positive effects, ultimately leading to lowered blood pressure and improved overall physical well-being. Yoga, another spiritual practice, weaves together movement, breath, and mindfulness. As we flow through yoga postures, we not only strengthen our physical bodies but also delve into a profound connection with our inner selves. The result is a sense of calm and equilibrium that extends beyond the yoga mat. This equilibrium, in turn, contributes to reducing stress and promoting physical health.

Spirituality imparts a sense of purpose and meaning to life. It guides individuals toward a greater understanding of themselves and their place in the universe. This sense of purpose becomes a potent catalyst for the body's natural healing processes. When we believe that our lives have purpose and meaning, our bodies respond with enhanced resilience and vitality. This belief acts as a beacon, guiding our bodies towards healing and recovery during times of illness or adversity.

In summary, spirituality serves as a profound framework for understanding the intricate connection between the mind and body. It offers a unique perspective that emphasizes the inseparable nature of mental, emotional, and physical well-being. Through practices like meditation and yoga, individuals can harness the power of spirituality to reduce stress, lower blood pressure, and enhance their overall physical health. Furthermore, the sense of purpose and meaning derived from spiritual beliefs acts as a potent elixir, stimulating the body's innate healing mechanisms. In embracing spirituality, we embark on a holistic journey toward wellness, where the mind and body are harmoniously united in their pursuit of health and happiness.

Spirituality in Coping with Adversity:

Life's journey is riddled with challenges and adversities. Spirituality acts as a lantern in the dark, providing hope and resilience. It helps individuals make sense of suffering, offering a framework to navigate pain and loss. This coping mechanism can be particularly invaluable during times of grief or illness, as it fosters acceptance and a sense of transcendence. One of the central roles of spirituality in coping with adversity is its ability to provide individuals with a sense of purpose and meaning. It allows individuals to view suffering not as an arbitrary and meaningless aspect of life but as a part of a larger, interconnected narrative. This sense of purpose can instill hope and motivate individuals to persevere through difficult times, believing that their experiences contribute to a greater purpose.

Spirituality also offers a framework for navigating the complex emotions that often accompany adversity. When individuals face grief, loss, or illness, they can turn to their spiritual beliefs to find comfort and understanding. For example, many religious and spiritual traditions emphasize concepts like redemption, forgiveness, and the idea of a divine plan. These beliefs can provide solace and help individuals make sense of their suffering, alleviating feelings of confusion and despair.

Moreover, spirituality can foster acceptance and resilience in the face of adversity. It encourages individuals to confront their challenges with courage and equanimity. Through spiritual practices such as meditation, prayer, or mindfulness, individuals can find inner peace and tranquility, even amidst turmoil. This inner peace can help reduce stress, anxiety, and depression, promoting emotional well-being.

In times of adversity, spirituality can also serve as a source of community and support. Places of worship, spiritual gatherings, and religious communities often provide a sense of belonging and connection. The support of like-minded individuals who share similar beliefs and values can be a tremendous source of strength and encouragement during difficult times Another notable aspect of spirituality in adversity is its capacity to offer a sense of transcendence. Many spiritual traditions teach that there is more to life than the material world, and adversity can be seen as an opportunity for personal growth and spiritual transformation. This perspective encourages individuals to look beyond their immediate circumstances and seek a higher purpose or connection with the divine. Spirituality plays a vital role in helping individuals cope with adversity by offering hope, meaning, acceptance, and resilience. It provides a framework to navigate the complexities of suffering and serves as a source of strength during times of grief, loss, or illness. While the specifics of spiritual beliefs and practices vary widely, the common thread is the capacity of spirituality to illuminate the path through life's darkest moments, ultimately helping individuals find light and purpose in the face of adversity.

The Interplay of Culture and Spirituality:

Cultural context plays a significant role in shaping an individual's spirituality. Every culture has its unique rituals, symbols, and belief systems that intertwine with spirituality. Recognizing and respecting this diversity is essential when studying spirituality's influence on well-being, as it allows for a nuanced understanding of its impact across different societies and communities.

Spirituality, as a deeply personal and multifaceted facet of human existence, exerts a profound influence on well-being. It fosters emotional resilience, cultivates mental clarity, and nurtures physical health. Moreover, it provides solace in times of adversity and a sense of purpose in the face of life's mysteries. To fully appreciate its impact, one must acknowledge the interplay of culture and spirituality, recognizing that the tapestry of well-being is richly woven with threads of spirituality, each unique and distinct.

Chapter 7

Environmental Factors in Holistic Health

Introduction:

Holistic health is an approach that considers the entire person, emphasizing the connection between mind, body, and spirit. While factors such as diet, exercise, and mental well-being are often at the forefront of holistic health discussions, the environment plays a pivotal and often underestimated role in shaping our overall well-being. This write-up explores the intricate relationship between environmental factors and holistic health, highlighting their unique and distinct impact on our physical, mental, and emotional health.

I. Air Quality: Breathing Life into Holistic Health

Clean air is fundamental to our existence, yet it's often taken for granted. Poor air quality, laden with pollutants, can lead to respiratory diseases, allergies, and stress. The quality of the air we breathe directly affects our physical well-being and has a profound influence on our mental clarity and emotional balance. In the grand symphony of existence, the air we breathe plays a pivotal role, like the silent conductor of an orchestra. It orchestrates our vitality, impacts our very essence, yet, all too often, it remains unnoticed, taken for granted like the quiet background music of our lives. The undeniable truth is that clean air is not just a luxury; it is a fundamental prerequisite for our survival and well-being.

Imagine for a moment, a world where the air is thick with pollutants, where every inhalation fills your lungs with microscopic adversaries, where the very essence of life becomes a health hazard. This is the grim reality faced by many in regions plagued by poor air quality. The consequences of this silent assailant are manifold and far-reaching. At the forefront of this battlefield are our respiratory systems, the unsung heroes tirelessly processing the air we breathe. When this air is tainted with pollutants, it triggers a chain reaction within our bodies. The inhalation of particulate matter, noxious gases, and harmful chemicals can lead to a host of respiratory diseases, each with its own set of dire consequences. Conditions such as asthma, bronchitis, and chronic obstructive pulmonary disease (COPD) become more prevalent and severe in areas with poor air quality. Our lungs, the delicate bellows of our existence, bear the brunt of this environmental assault.

Yet, the impact of air quality extends beyond the confines of our respiratory systems. It reaches deep into the fibers of our being, affecting not only our physical health but also our mental and emotional states. Imagine standing in a pristine forest, inhaling the crisp, clean air, and feeling an overwhelming sense of tranquility and rejuvenation. Contrast this with the experience of walking through a smog-choked cityscape, where every breath is a laborious effort, and the psychological toll is palpable. Clean air, like a soothing balm for the mind, has a profound influence on our mental clarity and emotional balance. Research has shown a clear link between air quality and cognitive function. When we breathe clean, oxygen-rich air, our brains receive the nourishment they need to function optimally. Conversely, polluted air can impair cognitive abilities, leading to decreased productivity, memory problems, and even mood disorders.

Moreover, the emotional resonance of air quality cannot be overstated. Picture the joy of a clear, sunny day where the sky is an endless blue canvas, versus the gloom and unease that accompanies days when smog obscures the sun. The impact on our emotional well-being is undeniable. Poor air quality can contribute to stress, anxiety, and even depression, creating a vicious cycle where compromised mental health further undermines physical health.

The quality of the air we breathe is an intricate thread woven into the tapestry of our holistic health. It affects not only our lungs but also our minds and hearts. It's a testament to the interconnectedness of our existence, where the environment we inhabit intimately shapes our well-being. To truly appreciate the significance of air quality is to acknowledge it as a cornerstone of our lives. It is the unseen force that breathes life into holistic health, a reminder that in the grand narrative of existence, every breath counts, and the quality of each inhalation shapes our journey toward well-being and balance. Thus, let us not take the gift of clean air for granted, but instead, embrace it as the vital elixir of life it truly is.

II. Natural Spaces: The Healing Power of Nature

Access to natural environments, such as parks and forests, has been linked to reduced stress, improved mood, and enhanced cognitive function. Nature provides a sanctuary for the mind and body, allowing us to reconnect with our inner selves and find solace in its serenity. The relationship between nature and holistic health underscores the importance of green spaces in our urban landscapes.

The allure of nature's embrace transcends the mere aesthetic appeal of parks and forests; it delves into the profound realm of emotional and physiological healing. Within the verdant tapestry of our natural landscapes, there exists an astonishing remedy for the tumultuous rhythms of modern life. In these tranquil sanctuaries, where the rustling leaves compose a soothing symphony, and the dappling sunlight paints patterns of tranquility, we discover more than just a respite from urban chaos. Nature unveils itself as a holistic healer, extending its therapeutic touch to our very core. The subtle symphony of chirping birds and babbling brooks serves as a melodic balm for our frayed nerves, effortlessly melting away the stress that clings to us like an unwanted shadow. In the midst of this lush serenity, our minds find respite, and the burdens of daily life slip away like forgotten troubles. We stand on the threshold of a cognitive renaissance, where creativity flourishes, and clarity of thought reigns supreme. But it's not just our minds that nature nurtures; it's our souls as well. In these pristine landscapes, we rediscover a connection with our inner selves, long overshadowed by the hustle and bustle of our urban existence. There, amidst the towering trees and gentle murmurs of the wind, we find solace. Nature becomes the mirror that reflects our true essence, offering us a chance to rediscover who we are beneath the layers of modernity. The profound relationship between natural spaces and holistic health underscores a fundamental truth: in our increasingly urbanized world, the importance of green havens cannot be overstated. They are not mere luxuries but essential sanctuaries for our well-being. As we venture into the heart of these green oases, we embark on a journey of rediscovery, where nature's embrace becomes the path to healing, rejuvenation, and a deeper connection to ourselves and the world around us.

III. Chemical Exposures: Unseen Threats to Well-Being

Our daily lives expose us to a multitude of chemicals found in food, personal care products, and the environment. Some of these chemicals, like pesticides and synthetic additives, can disrupt our hormonal balance and immune system, contributing to chronic health issues. Recognizing and minimizing chemical exposures is crucial for holistic health. In the intricate tapestry of our existence, we are unwittingly entwined with an array of chemical substances, woven seamlessly into our daily lives. These unseen agents pervade not only our food but also our personal care products and the very air we breathe, forming an invisible web that poses a surreptitious threat to our well-being.

Amongst these clandestine compounds, a disquieting faction stands out – pesticides and synthetic additives. These elusive intruders have the power to infiltrate our bodies, camouflaging their impact until it's too late. They work silently, disrupting the delicate symphony of our hormonal balance and the sentinel fortifications of our immune system. It's a nefarious dance, leading to the insidious rise of chronic health issues that lurk beneath the surface of our awareness. Recognizing the true extent of this threat is not only paramount but also a moral obligation to our holistic health. It demands that we unveil these chemical specters, shining a light on their shadowy presence. By doing so, we empower ourselves to take action, to mitigate the dangers they pose, and ultimately to reclaim sovereignty over our well-being. This is a call to arms, an awakening to the fact that the unseen dangers of chemical exposures are as potent as they are elusive. Only by acknowledging their existence and striving to minimize our interaction with them can we hope to safeguard our health in a world where these hidden adversaries lurk around every corner."

IV. Noise Pollution: The Unheard Culprit

Noise pollution can disrupt sleep patterns, increase stress levels, and even contribute to heart disease. Its adverse effects on mental and emotional well-being are often overlooked. Quiet, peaceful environments are essential for promoting inner harmony and holistic health. Noise pollution, often considered the silent saboteur of our well-being, stealthily infiltrates our lives with consequences that extend far beyond mere annoyance. While it's commonly recognized for disturbing our sleep patterns, elevating stress levels, and even potentially playing a role in the development of heart disease, its insidious effects on our mental and emotional well-being remain largely unheard. In a world bustling with incessant clamor, the profound toll noise pollution exacts on our inner harmony is often overshadowed by its more visible manifestations. Beyond the restless nights and frayed nerves lies a deeper layer of impact.

Noise pollution infiltrates our psyche, subtly eroding our sense of calm, and gradually chipping away at our emotional resilience. Imagine a world where the serenity of silence is no longer a luxury but a necessity. In this context, quiet, peaceful environments become not just a luxury, but an essential component of our holistic health. They offer us refuge from the relentless cacophony of modern life, providing a haven where our minds can recharge, our emotions can find balance, and our spirits can reconnect with the tranquility that nature intended. To truly understand the scope of noise pollution's influence, we must not merely focus on its overt disruptions but delve deeper into the subtle erosion of our mental and emotional well-being. It's time to acknowledge the unheard culprit and work towards restoring the quietude our souls desperately crave."

V. Climate Change: The Global Health Challenge

Climate change is no longer just an environmental concern; it's a holistic health crisis. Rising temperatures, extreme weather events, and food insecurity are all consequences that directly impact our well-being. Addressing climate change is not only an ecological imperative but a holistic health necessity. Climate change has transformed from being solely an environmental issue into a comprehensive health crisis that affects every facet of human well-being. The repercussions of this phenomenon extend far beyond rising temperatures and the depletion of polar ice caps; they infiltrate our daily lives, pose an existential threat to our health, and demand urgent and transformative action. One of the most immediate and pressing concerns in the context of climate change is the rise in global temperatures. As the Earth's average temperature continues to climb, we witness a surge in the frequency and intensity of heatwaves. Prolonged exposure to extreme heat not only jeopardizes our physical health by increasing the risk of heat-related illnesses, but it also exacerbates pre-existing conditions, such as cardiovascular diseases and respiratory problems. Vulnerable populations, including the elderly and those with limited access to cooling resources, bear the brunt of these health impacts.

Climate change is intrinsically linked to the occurrence of extreme weather events. Hurricanes, floods, wildfires, and droughts are becoming more frequent and severe due to shifting weather patterns. These events result in immediate injuries and fatalities, but their aftermath often gives rise to longer-term health crises. Displaced populations face the risk of infectious disease outbreaks in crowded shelters, and disrupted healthcare infrastructure hampers the delivery of essential medical services. Food security is another critical facet of the climate change and health nexus. Rising temperatures and altered precipitation patterns affect crop yields and threaten the global food supply. Reduced access to nutritious food can lead to malnutrition and foodborne diseases, particularly in impoverished regions where resources are already scarce. This not only impacts physical health but also compromises cognitive development in children, perpetuating a cycle of poverty and ill health.

Addressing climate change is not merely an environmental endeavor; it is a prerequisite for safeguarding public health on a global scale. Tackling this challenge necessitates comprehensive strategies that go beyond reducing greenhouse gas emissions. It involves implementing adaptive measures to protect vulnerable communities, fortifying healthcare systems to respond to climate-related emergencies, and investing in research to better understand the complex interplay between climate change and health. Climate change has evolved into a global health crisis with far-reaching consequences. From the immediate threats of heatwaves and extreme weather events to the insidious impacts on food security and nutrition, the health of individuals and communities is intricately intertwined with the changing climate. Recognizing this interconnectedness is the first step toward forging a sustainable and healthier future for all. The time for action is now, as mitigating climate change is not only an environmental imperative but a matter of life and well-being for generations to come.

VI. The Built Environment: Shaping Health and Well-Being

Our homes, workplaces, and communities have a profound impact on our holistic health. Access to safe, walkable neighborhoods, green architecture, and spaces that foster social connections all contribute to a healthier and more balanced life.

In our quest for holistic health, we must recognize that our well-being is intricately linked to the environment that surrounds us. The air we breathe, the natural spaces we inhabit, the chemicals we encounter, the sounds we hear, and the changing climate all play unique and distinct roles in shaping our health. To achieve true holistic health, we must prioritize the protection and nurturing of our environment, for in doing so, we simultaneously nurture our minds, bodies, and spirits.

Chapter 8

Crafting Your Holistic Health Plan: A Personalized Journey

In a world where wellness is increasingly paramount, the journey towards holistic health has become a unique and deeply personal endeavor. "Crafting Your Holistic Health Plan: A Personalized Journey" is not just a guide; it's an invitation to embark on a transformative odyssey towards a healthier and more balanced life. The foundation of this journey lies in the understanding that health isn't solely the absence of illness; it's a harmonious equilibrium of mind, body, and spirit. Your personalized roadmap to holistic health is a symphony of individualized choices, weaving together diverse elements to create a life that resonates with vitality.

Begin with introspection, for self-awareness is the compass of your voyage. Assess your physical, emotional, and mental states honestly. What are your strengths, weaknesses, and aspirations? Identify the unique tapestry of your life, the threads of habits, routines, and experiences that have shaped you.

Next, engage in the art of nourishment. Explore whole, nutritious foods that fuel not only your body but also your spirit. Delight in the vibrant flavors of nature's bounty, understanding that food is not just sustenance but a source of joy and vitality. As you progress, delve into the world of movement. Craft an exercise regimen that dances with your passions, whether it's yoga under the morning sun, the rhythmic beats of a dance class, or the serenity of a forest hike. Movement isn't a chore; it's a celebration of your body's capabilities.

Mindfulness becomes your companion on this odyssey. Embrace meditation, deep breathing, or mindfulness practices that center your thoughts and emotions. In the quiet moments, you discover the power of the present, untangling the threads of stress and anxiety that may have held you back. Nurture your relationships, for they are the threads connecting you to the world. Cultivate connections that uplift, support, and inspire you. Remember that social well-being is an essential facet of holistic health.

Sleep, like a gentle lullaby, rejuvenates your spirit. Craft a sleep ritual that honors your body's need for rest, granting you the energy to embrace each day with vigor. The environment you inhabit plays a crucial role in your well-being. Embrace sustainability and eco-conscious choices, for a healthy planet mirrors a healthy life.

Ultimately, crafting your holistic health plan is an ongoing process. It's not a rigid blueprint but a flexible canvas, adapting to the seasons of your life. Embrace your unique journey, acknowledging that setbacks are part of the mosaic, not the end of the road. In "Crafting Your Holistic Health Plan: A Personalized Journey," you become the artist of your well-being, weaving together the threads of nutrition, movement, mindfulness, relationships, sleep, and environment into a masterpiece of vitality. This is your journey, your story, and your path to a life of lasting health and profound well-being.

Crafting a holistic health plan involves considering your physical, mental, and emotional well-being. Here are steps to create one:

Self-Assessment:

Reflect on your current health status, including physical, mental, and emotional aspects.

Identify areas that need improvement or attention.

Set Clear Goals:

Define specific, measurable, achievable, relevant, and time-bound (SMART) goals for each aspect of your health.

Nutrition:

Develop a balanced diet rich in whole foods, fruits, vegetables, and lean proteins. Take into account your dietary limitations or any allergies you may possess.

Exercise:

Create a fitness routine that includes cardiovascular, strength training, and flexibility exercises. Set a realistic schedule and gradually increase intensity.

Sleep:

Prioritize quality sleep by establishing a consistent sleep schedule and creating a comfortable sleep environment.

Stress Management:

Practice relaxation techniques like meditation, deep breathing, or yoga.

Identify stressors and work on coping strategies.

Mental Health:

Seek professional help if needed. Prioritize self-care and engage in activities that bring you joy and relaxation.

Emotional Well-being:

Build a support system of friends and family.

Explore hobbies and activities that fulfill you emotionally.

Preventive Care:

Schedule regular check-ups with healthcare professionals.

Stay up-to-date with vaccinations and screenings.

Holistic Therapies:

Consider alternative therapies such as acupuncture, massage, or aromatherapy if they align with your beliefs.

Monitoring and Adjusting:

Regularly assess your progress towards your goals. Modify your strategy as required to accommodate evolving situation.

Accountability:

Share your plan with a trusted friend or partner who can help keep you accountable.

Mindfulness:

Practice mindfulness to stay in tune with your body's signals and adjust your plan accordingly.

Education:

Stay informed about health-related topics through reputable sources.

Holistic Approach:

Recognize the interconnectedness of your physical, mental, and emotional health. Seek equilibrium in every facet of your existence. Remember that crafting a holistic health plan is a personal journey, and it may evolve over time as your needs and circumstances change. Consulting with healthcare professionals, nutritionists, and mental health experts can provide valuable guidance.